Healing Hearts: How Our Striking Nurses Deserve Fair Wages and Benefits

Unmasking the Unjust Treatment of Nursing Professionals: Why They Deserve Fair Pay and Respect

By

Renee E. Hills

Table of contents

INTRODUCTION

The strike nurse had been working in the same hospital for over 20 years. She was a dedicated and hardworking nurse, but she was often overlooked and underpaid. She had been fighting for better wages and working conditions since she started but had made little progress.

One day, the strike nurse heard about a new bill that had been introduced by a local politician. It proposed that strike nurses be paid a fair wage for their hard work and dedication. The strike nurse was thrilled and quickly began organizing her colleagues to support the bill.

The strike nurse and her colleagues held protests, marched in parades, and met with local politicians to show their support for the bill. After months of hard work, the bill was finally passed, and the strike nurse and her colleagues were finally given the pay they deserved.

The strike nurse was overjoyed. She had worked hard for years and finally achieved her goal of being paid fairly for her work. She was proud of her accomplishments and was happy to know that future strike nurses would benefit from her efforts. The strike nurse was now able to provide for her family and continue to care for her patients with the respect and financial security she deserved.

The strike nurse was used to not being paid fairly. She had been working in the same hospital for over 20 years and had been fighting for better wages and working conditions since she started. Despite her dedication and hard work, she was often overlooked and underpaid. She was determined to make a difference, so she began organizing her colleagues to support a new bill that proposed strike nurses be paid a fair wage.

After months of hard work and dedication, the bill was finally passed and the strike nurse and her colleagues were finally given the pay they deserved. The strike nurse was relieved and happy to know that future strike nurses would benefit from her efforts. She was proud of her accomplishments and was now able to provide for her family and continue to care for her patients with the respect and financial security she deserved.

The government should ensure that all nurses are paid fairly for their hard work and dedication. This includes strike nurses, who are often overlooked and are not paid a wage that reflects the value of their work. The government should work with employers to ensure that all nurses are paid a fair wage and that their working conditions are safe and healthy. Furthermore, the government should continue to introduce legislation that will ensure that strike nurses are paid a wage that reflects the value of their work. This will help to ensure that nurses are able to provide for their families and receive the respect they deserve.

CHAPTER ONE:Meaning of nurse

A nurse is a trained healthcare professional who provides preventative care, treatment, and health education to individuals and families. Nurses work in many different settings, including hospitals, nursing homes, schools, and other health care centers. They may also work in private practice, providing health services to patients in their homes or offices. A nurse is responsible for assessing patient needs and providing appropriate care, including physical and emotional support, as well as monitoring patient progress and updating medical records. Nurses also play an important role in public health initiatives, providing information and resources to the community. Nurses must possess a broad knowledge of health care, as well as excellent communication and interpersonal skills in order to be successful in their role. They must also be compassionate and empathetic, understanding the importance of treating each patient with respect and dignity.

Nursing is one of the oldest and most respected professions in healthcare. Nurses provide patient care, teach patients and the public about various health conditions, and provide advice and emotional support to patients and their families. Nurses work in a variety of settings, including hospitals, nursing homes, clinics, doctor's offices, and community health organizations.

Nurses must have excellent communication and organizational skills, as well as knowledge of medical procedures and treatments. To become a nurse, individuals must complete an accredited nursing program, which can include an associate's or bachelor's degree program, or a diploma program. After completing their studies, nurses must obtain a nursing license in order to practice.

Nurses have a variety of duties, including taking medical histories, performing physical exams, administering medications, and providing patient education. They must also be able to recognize signs and symptoms of illnesses, and provide assistance to physicians during medical procedures.

Nurses must also be able to provide emotional support to patients and their families, and be able to work as part of a healthcare team. Nurses must also be knowledgeable about safety regulations, infection control, and other legal and ethical issues.

Nurses also have the opportunity to specialize in a particular area of healthcare, such as pediatrics, geriatrics, oncology, or emergency medicine. Nurses also have the opportunity to pursue additional certifications and degrees, such as a master's degree in nursing or a doctorate in nursing practice.

As the coronavirus pandemic continues to spread across the world, healthcare workers are on the front lines, battling the virus and caring for those who have been infected. Nurses, in particular, are the backbone of the healthcare system and are working tirelessly to keep us safe. They are risking their lives every day, yet they are not being adequately compensated for their hard work. It is time for governments and healthcare organizations to recognize the importance of nurses and to provide them with fair wages and benefits.

Nurses are essential to the healthcare system, providing direct patient care and vital support to doctors. They are often the first line of defense in a medical emergency, and they are responsible for providing important medical advice and treatments to patients. Nurses are also responsible for monitoring patient progress and providing emotional support to both patients and their families.

The work that nurses do is essential and often physically and emotionally demanding. They must be on call 24 hours a day, seven days a week, often with little rest. Despite the sacrifices they make, nurses are not being adequately compensated for the critical work they do. Many nurses are underpaid and lack access to basic benefits such as health insurance and retirement plans.

It is important for governments and healthcare organizations to recognize the valuable contributions that nurses make to society and to ensure that they are fairly compensated for their hard work. Nurses should be provided with livable wages and benefits that will help them support their families and provide for their own future. This is especially important in light of the coronavirus pandemic, where nurses are on the front lines providing critical care and support.

In addition to providing nurses with fair wages and benefits, healthcare organizations must also ensure that they are given proper recognition and respect. Nurses should be given a seat at the table when it comes to making decisions about healthcare policy and the provision of care. This will ensure that their voices are heard and that their valuable input is taken into account.

It is time for governments and healthcare organizations to recognize the vital role that nurses play in the healthcare system and to ensure that they are fairly compensated for their hard work. This is essential for the well-being of both patients and nurses, and it is a critical step towards creating a healthier and more equitable healthcare system.

CHAPTER TWO: Advantages and Important of How Our Striking Nurses Deserve Fair Wages and Benefits

1. Improved Patient Care: Nurses are the backbone of any healthcare system, and providing them with fair wages and benefits will lead to improved patient care.

2. Job Satisfaction: Providing nurses with fair wages and benefits will help create a sense of job satisfaction and increase morale, leading to a happier and more productive workforce.

3. Financial Security: Fair wages and benefits will ensure that nurses have

financial security so they can plan for their future and the future of their families.

4. Increased Retention: Providing fair wages and benefits will help retain experienced nurses, leading to better continuity of care and improved patient outcomes.

5. Improved Recruitment: Offering fair wages and benefits will make the nursing profession more attractive to potential recruits, leading to higher quality and more experienced staff.

6. Professional Development: Fair wages and benefits will allow nurses to invest in their professional development, helping them to stay up to date with the latest advances in healthcare.

7. Respect: Providing fair wages and benefits to nurses shows them that their hard work and dedication is respected and valued by their employers.

8. Cost Savings: Providing nurses with fair wages and benefits can lead to cost savings in the long term, as nurses are less likely to require time off due to financial stress or burnout.

Benefits of our nurses

1. Provide patient-centered care
2. Promote health and wellness
3. Monitor patient health and provide education
4. Advocate for patients
5. Administer medication and treatments
6. Coordinate care plans with other health professionals
7. Address acute and chronic physical, mental and emotional health needs
8. Perform diagnostic tests, collect and analyze results
9. Identify, prevent and treat diseases
10. Administer intravenous fluids, medications and nutrition

11. Educate patients and families about health maintenance
12. Monitor vital signs, respond to changes and alert physicians
13. Maintain accurate medical records and reports
14. Provide emotional support and comfort to patients and families
15. Coordinate discharge planning and follow-up care
16. Manage patient care budgets
17. Assess, plan, implement and evaluate nursing care
18. Participate in research and quality improvement initiatives
19. Foster positive relationships with patients and families
20. Promote healthy lifestyles and preventive care strategies

CHAPTER THREE: List of important nurses across the whole world

1. Florence Nightingale – The founder of modern nursing, Florence Nightingale was a pioneering nurse who helped revolutionize the field through her work in hospitals, the development of educational institutions, and her tireless efforts to improve public health.

2. Mary Seacole – A Jamaican-born nurse, Mary Seacole was a pioneering nurse who self-funded her own trip to the Crimean War to provide medical care to British soldiers.

3. Clara Barton – Known as the "Angel of the Battlefield," Clara Barton was an American nurse and founder of the American Red Cross.

4. Dorothea Dix – An American social reformer, Dorothea Dix was a pioneer in the area of mental health care and opened the first public mental health hospital in the United States.

5. Linda Richards – The first professionally trained American nurse, Linda Richards was an innovator in the field of nursing and opened the first nursing school in the United States.

6. Virginia Avenel Henderson – An American nurse and theorist, Virginia Avenel Henderson was an influential figure in the development of modern nursing practice.

7. Jessie Scales – An American nurse who served in World War I, Jessie Scales was the first African-American nurse to serve in the U.S. Army.

8. Edith Cavell – A British nurse who served in World War I, Edith Cavell was a pioneering nurse who pushed for better care of wounded soldiers and was famously executed by the Germans for helping Allied soldiers escape.

9. Mabel Keaton Staupers – An African-American nurse and civil rights activist, Mabel Keaton Staupers fought for the inclusion of African-American nurses in the U.S. military and nursing education.

10. Margaret Sanger – A nurse and birth control activist, Margaret Sanger was an influential figure in the development of modern reproductive health care and was a key figure in the movement for women's rights.

11. Lucille Teasdale – A Canadian surgeon and humanitarian, Lucille Teasdale was the first international aid worker to work in

Africa and was dedicated to improving health care in war-torn countries.

12. Lillian Wald – An American nurse and social reformer, Lillian Wald was a pioneer in public health and the founder of the Henry Street Settlement in New York City.

13. Elizabeth Kenny – An Australian nurse who revolution ized the treatment of polio, Elizabeth Kenny was a pioneering nurse who developed the "Sister Kenny" treatment for polio.

14. Louise McManus – An American nurse and epidemiologist, Louise McManus was a pioneer in the field of public health and was one of the first nurses to work in the field of epidemiology.

15. Clara Maass – An American nurse who served in World War I, Clara Maass was a pioneering nurse who selflessly volunteered

to be infected with yellow fever in order to study the disease.

16. Mary Eliza Mahoney – The first African-American professional nurse in the United States, Mary Eliza Mahoney was an important figure in the civil rights movement.

17. Mary Breckinridge – An American nurse and midwife, Mary Breckinridge was a pioneer in the field of public health and founded the Frontier Nursing Service.

18. Lavinia Dock – An American nurse and social reformer, Lavinia Dock was a pioneer in the field of nursing education and was a leader in the effort to modernize nursing practices.

19. Mary Adelaide Nutting – Known as the "Mother of Nursing Education," Mary Adelaide Nutting was an influential figure

in the development of modern nursing education.

20. Doris Buffet – An American nurse and philanthropist, Doris Buffet was a pioneer in the field of public health and was the first female president of the American Red Cross.

CHAPTER FOUR: Roles of nurses in hospital

1. Provide patient care: Nurses are responsible for providing patient care to those in the hospital. This includes taking vital signs, administering medication, providing wound care, providing emotional support, and providing education to patients and families.

2. Collaborate with other healthcare professionals: Nurses work with physicians, pharmacists, physical therapists, and other healthcare professionals to ensure that all aspects of the patient's care are addressed.

3. Serve as patient advocates: Nurses serve as patient advocates and ensure that the patient's wishes and rights are respected.

4. Develop and implement patient care plans: Nurses develop and implement patient care plans that are tailored to the individual needs of the patient.

5. Coordinate patient discharge: Nurses coordinate patient discharge from the hospital and ensure that the patient has the resources and support needed to continue care at home.

6. Administer treatments: Nurses administer treatments such as IVs, injections, and wound care.

7. Monitor patient progress: Nurses monitor the progress of patients and communicate changes in condition to other healthcare professionals.

8. Educate patients and families: Nurses provide education to patients and families about their diagnosis, treatment,

medications, and other aspects of their care.

CHAPTER FIVE: Types of nurses

There are a variety of types of nurses, each with their own unique skills and responsibilities.

1. Registered Nurses (RNs): Registered nurses are the most common type of nurse. They provide direct patient care, such as assessing patients' health, administering medications, and monitoring vital signs. RNs also educate patients and the public about health care.

2. Certified Nurse Assistants (CNAs): CNAs provide basic nursing care, such as helping patients with activities of daily living, such as bathing and dressing.

3. Licensed Practical Nurses (LPNs): LPNs provide basic nursing care and can also

evaluate patients' responses to treatments and medications.

4. Advanced Practice Registered Nurses (APRNs): APRNs are highly educated and experienced nurses who provide specialized care, such as prescribing medications, treating diseases, and performing procedures.

5. Nurse Practitioners (NPs): NPs are advanced practice registered nurses with additional education and expertise in a particular field, such as pediatrics or geriatrics.

6. Clinical Nurse Specialists (CNSs): CNSs are advanced practice registered nurses who specialize in a specific area of nursing, such as mental health

7. Nurse Anesthetists (CRNAs): CRNAs are advanced practice registered nurses who administer anesthesia and other

medications to patients before, during, and after medical procedures.

8. Nurse Midwives: Nurse midwives are advanced practice registered nurses who specialize in providing care to pregnant women and delivering babies.

9. Nursing Instructors: Nursing instructors are experienced nurses who teach nursing students in a classroom or clinical setting.

10. Nurse Managers: Nurse managers are experienced registered nurses who oversee the day-to-day operations of a nursing unit or department.

CHAPTER SIX: Qualities of Nurses

Nurses have a number of important qualities that make them an invaluable component of the healthcare system.

First and foremost, nurses have excellent communication skills. They need to be able to effectively communicate with patients, their families, and other healthcare professionals in order to provide the best care. This includes being able to listen carefully and provide clear information in an understandable manner.

Nurses also need to be highly organized in order to ensure that all of their patients' needs are being met. They must be able to prioritize tasks and manage their time wisely.

Additionally, nurses must possess a high level of compassion and empathy. Caring for patients can be emotionally demanding, so nurses need to be able to show understanding and support.

Finally, nurses must have strong problem-solving skills. As they often face unpredictable situations, nurses need to be able to quickly assess a situation and find the best solution.

All of these qualities make nurses essential members of the healthcare team and invaluable to the patients they care for.

Paying our nurses fairly

Nurses are essential members of the healthcare system. They provide crucial medical care and support to patients in need. It is therefore important to ensure that nurses are paid fairly for their work.

Fair wages are necessary to ensure that nurses can afford to live comfortably and adequately provide for their families. Fair wages also provide nurses with the financial stability and security they need to continue providing quality care to their patients.

Fair wages also encourage nurses to remain in the profession and provide incentive for them to continue learning and growing in their field. Without fair wages, nurses may be discouraged from continuing to practice and instead choose to pursue other opportunities. This could lead to a shortage of qualified nurses and a decrease in the quality of care patients receive. Fair wages also help to attract new nurses to the profession, which is necessary to meet the growing demand for healthcare services.

Finally, fair wages are important to ensure that nurses are valued and respected for the important work they do. Nurses provide an invaluable service to their patients and their communities, and they should be justly compensated for their hard work and dedication. Fair wages also show nurses that their work is appreciated and valued.

In short, nurses need to be paid fairly in order to ensure that they are able to continue providing quality care to their patients, that they remain motivated to do their best work, and that they are able to provide for themselves and their families. Fair pay is essential for the healthcare system to remain strong, and nurses deserve to be justly compensated for the important work that they do.

CHAPTER SEVEN: Responsibility of nurses

Nurses are responsible for providing direct patient care and ensuring that the patient receives the best possible care. This includes assessing the patient's condition and medical needs, administering medications and treatments, monitoring vital signs, and providing emotional support and education to the patient and their family. Nurses must also be responsible for maintaining accurate patient records and working collaboratively with other healthcare professionals to coordinate a course of treatment. Additionally, nurses are responsible for staying up to date on the latest medical advancements and techniques. They must also adhere to strict ethical and legal standards when caring for patients. In some cases, nurses may also be responsible for developing and coordinating care plans, advocating for patients, and educating the public on health and wellness.

List of responsibility of nurses are ;

1. Administering medication and treatments as prescribed by physicians.
2. Observing and recording patient behavior.
3. Assisting patients with daily activities.
4. Educating patients and their families about health conditions.
5. Assessing patient health by interviewing patients and performing physical examinations.
6. Developing care plans for individual patients.
7. Monitoring and reporting patient progress to physicians.
8. Coordinating patient care with other health care professionals.
9. Responding to life-saving situations, using nursing standards and protocols.

10. Maintaining patient confidentiality and adhering to HIPAA regulations.

Things to know before becoming a nurse

1. Be prepared to work long hours and days, often with little sleep.
2. Understand patient confidentiality and HIPAA laws.
3. Have strong communication skills.
4. Learn how to multitask.
5. Have empathy and compassion for your patients.
6. Develop a thick skin and a strong sense of resilience.
7. Have a strong work ethic.
8. Have a basic understanding of common medical terminology.
9. Be organized and detail-oriented.
10. Have the ability to think quickly and make decisions in high-pressure situations.

11. Stay up-to-date on the latest medical advancements.
12. Have a basic knowledge of anatomy and physiology.
13. Become familiar with common medications and treatments.
14. Learn how to properly document patient care.
15. Gain experience with medical equipment and supplies.
16. Have an understanding of insurance and billing procedures.
17. Be able to read and interpret lab results.
18. Understand how to prioritize tasks.
19. Have a basic understanding of medical coding.
20. Be able to work well with a variety of personnel.

CHAPTER EIGHT: Why are attendants striking?

The Illustrious School of Nursing (RCN) balloted its individuals over modern activity in a disagreement regarding pay. It has contended that low compensation is driving "constant understaffing" that seriously endangers patients and leaves nursing staff exhausted, coming up short on and underestimated.

Is there an emergency in the labor force?

The number of medical caretakers and birthing specialists enrolled to work in the UK has developed to a record level - 771,445 were on the Nursing and Birthing assistance Gathering register in September. However, separate figures from NHS Computerized show there were a record 47,496 full-time comparable nursing opportunities in Britain toward the finish of September, addressing an opening pace of 11.9%.

What number of medical caretakers will be protesting?

Work MPs join medical caretakers on picket lines - attendants strike, as it worked out
Understand more
A huge number of medical caretakers are to participate - initially, it was guessed that up to 100,000 would strike however this figure changed due to the different "criticisms" that have happened lately where attendants have consented to offer particular types of assistance during strike days.

When will the strikes occur?

The strikes are planned for Thursday 15 December and Tuesday 20 December, albeit not all associations are partaking in the two days.

What occurs assuming I'm wiped out?

Individuals who need crisis or dire consideration will in any case find support. The strikes will influence different components of care however individuals will have been reached ahead of time to be recounted changes to arranged care and urged to go to arrangements except if they have been told in any case. GP medical procedures and drug stores will be running as expected.

What has the Regal School of Nursing requested?

The RCN requested a 12.5% salary raise in 2020. Some place during the debate it was guaranteed that medical caretakers needed a "5% above expansion rise" - probably when expansion was 7.5% or somewhere around there.

So what has been advertised?

A free compensation survey body suggested that most NHS staff on purported Plan for Change contracts are to be given a £1,400 ascend in pay. The Nuffield Trust has assessed that this is identical to a normal of 4.3% ascent for qualified attendants. The RCN has recently expressed that notwithstanding the current year's compensation grant, experienced medical caretakers are more terribly off by 20% in genuine terms due to progressive beneath expansion grants starting around 2010.

What has the public authority said?

The public authority acknowledged the suggestion by the compensation survey body and it has said that association requests are "not reasonable" in the ongoing monetary environment, saying each extra 1% compensation ascend for all Plan for Change staff would cost about £700m every year.

However, the compensation audit body assesses that each 1% salary raise adds about £500m to the Plan for Change take care of bill in Britain, £29.5m in Northern Ireland, and £37.5m in Ridges.

The Division of Well-being and that's what social Consideration said, utilizing October's RPI expansion information, a 5% above expansion rise would liken to a compensation ascent of 19.2%. It said that rising compensation for all staff on Plan for Change contracts - which likewise incorporates staff like maternity specialists, rescue vehicle laborers, watchmen, and cleaners - by 19.2%, rather than the current compensation grant, would cost "around an extra £10bn".

Authorities have said that this would hamper the NHS's endeavors in handling the record accumulation of care. Be that as it may, the RCN has not explicitly requested a 19.2% boost in compensation.

A different compensation offer has been made in Scotland.

What has the NHS said?

Authorities in Britain have said they might want to consider a goal to the debate to be soon as could be expected "yet pay is a matter for the public authority and the worker's guilds".

Where will the strikes occur?

Few out of every odd clinic will be impacted by strike activity. Here is the authority rundown of trusts and NHS associations partaking, delivered by the RCN:

Britain

East Midlands

Kettering general clinic NHS establishment trust

NHS Nottingham and Nottinghamshire ICB

Northamptonshire medical care NHS establishment trust

Nottingham College clinics NHS trust

Nottinghamshire medical care NHS establishment trust

Eastern

Cambridge College medical clinic NHS establishment trust

Cambridgeshire and Peterborough NHS establishment trust

Cambridgeshire People group Administrations NHS trust

Hertfordshire People group NHS trust

NHS Hertfordshire and West Essex ICB

Imperial Papworth emergency clinic NHS establishment trust

London

Extraordinary Ormond Road emergency clinic for Youngsters NHS establishment trust

Folks and St Thomas NHS establishment trust

Majestic School medical services NHS trust

NHS North Focal London ICB

Regal Marsden NHS establishment trust

North West

Birch Hello Youngsters' NHS establishment trust

Liverpool heart and chest clinic NHS establishment trust

Liverpool College Emergency clinics NHS establishment trust

Liverpool Ladies' NHS establishment trust

Mersey Care NHS establishment trust

The Clatterbridge Malignant growth Community NHS establishment trust

The Walton Place NHS establishment trust

Northern

Gateshead Wellbeing NHS establishment trust

Northumbria medical services NHS established a trust

The Newcastle Upon Tyne clinics NHS establishment trust

South East

Oxford Wellbeing NHS establishment trust

Oxford College clinics NHS establishment trust

Imperial Berkshire NHS establishment trust

Devon Organization NHS trust

Gloucestershire Wellbeing and Care NHS establishment trust

Gloucestershire emergency clinics NHS establishment trust

Incredible Western emergency clinics NHS establishment trust

NHS Shower, North East Somerset, Swindon and Wiltshire ICB (BSW Together)

NHS Devon ICB (One Devon)

NHS Gloucestershire ICB (One Gloucestershire)

North Bristol NHS Trust

Regal Devon College medical services NHS establishment trust

Regal Joined emergency clinics Shower NHS establishment trust

Torbay and South Devon NHS establishment trust

College emergency clinics Bristol and Weston NHS foundation trust

College clinics Plymouth NHS Trust

West Midlands

Birmingham Ladies' and Youngsters' NHS establishment trust

Herefordshire and Worcestershire Wellbeing and Care NHS Trust

NHS Birmingham and Solihull ICB (BSol ICB)

The Regal Muscular clinic NHS establishment trust

College emergency clinics Birmingham NHS establishment trust

Worcestershire Intense Emergency clinics NHS trust

Yorkshire and Humber

Bradford showing emergency clinics NHS establishment trust

Leeds people group medical care NHS trust

The Leeds showing medical clinics NHS trust

Public managers

Wellbeing Training Britain

NHS Britain

Northern Ireland

Belfast's well-being and social consideration trust

Northern well-being and social consideration trust

Western well-being and social consideration trust

Southern well-being and social consideration trust

South Eastern well-being and social consideration trust

Northern Ireland Practice and Schooling Committee

Business Administrations Association

Guideline and Quality Improvement Authority

Northern Ireland Blood Bonding Administration

General Wellbeing Organization

Northern Ireland rescue vehicle administration

Grains

Cardiff and Vale College wellbeing board

Powys Showing neighborhood wellbeing board

Welsh rescue vehicle administrations NHS trust central command

Hywel Dda College wellbeing board

Swansea Inlet College wellbeing board

Cwm Taf Morgannwg College wellbeing board

Betsi Cadwaladr College nearby the wellbeing board

Velindre NHS Trust

General Wellbeing Ridges

Wellbeing Instruction and Improvement Grains Wellbeing Authority

NHS Ridges Shared Administrations Organization

Advanced Wellbeing and Care Grains

A few NHS medical caretakers and emergency vehicle staff are striking over pay in the approach of Christmas.

Further modern activity is normal in the new year.

When are NHS staff striking?

Attendants

Individuals from the Regal School of Nursing (RCN) made a striking move briefly time on 20 December, having recently left on 15 December. The association has cautioned against additional strikes in the new year.

About a fourth of emergency clinics and local area groups in Britain were impacted, alongside all well-being sheets in Northern Ireland, and everything except one in Ribs. Turnout in the decision in favor of modern activity was excessively low in almost 50% of NHS confides in Britain for strikes to go for it.

The RCN in Scotland has said it will declare strike dates right on time one year from now after individuals dismissed a compensation bargain that would have seen the normal compensation ascend by 7.5%.

Imperial School of Birthing assistants (RCM) individuals in Scotland likewise dismissed the arrangement, and the association says it is thinking about conceivable modern activity.

Emergency vehicle staff

A few specialists in Britain and Grains are striking on 21 and 28 December.

The activity includes paramedics, control room staff, and backing laborers.

Individuals from the three principal rescue vehicle associations - Harmony, GMB and Join together - are partaking in the primary strike. GMB endorsers will strike in the future on 28 December.

The beginning times and lengths of the walkouts differ between emergency vehicle administrations, however, all will endure somewhere in the range of 12 and 24 hours. The East of Britain is the main help unaffected.

How might the NHS strikes affect patients?
Medical caretakers

Life-protecting treatment should be given. All medical attendants in escalated and crisis care are supposed to work.

Anybody who is genuinely sick or harmed ought to in any case call 999, or 111 for non-dire consideration.

Different administrations, like some disease medicines, might be somewhat staffed.

Routine consideration, like knee and hip substitutions, is probably going to be severely impacted.

Potential attendants could be pulled off picket lines to work assuming there are security concerns.

Emergency vehicle staff

The guidance stays for individuals to call 999 in a crisis.

All Classification 1 calls - the most hazardous circumstances, like heart failure - will be answered by a rescue vehicle.

Class 2 calls - for conditions that are serious yet not promptly dangerous, including a few strokes - probably won't be quickly gone to by crisis groups.

Class 3 calls -, for example, a lady in late-stage work - won't be focused on.

The people who have a fall, or experience other minor wounds which are not seen to be hazardous, are probably not going to get 999 consideration.

In such circumstances, a few NHS trusts are encouraging individuals to utilize their vehicles to get to the medical clinic or take a taxi.

Around 600 individuals from the military are because of taking on emergency vehicle driving jobs, and 150 staff will offer calculated help.

Why are medical attendants and emergency vehicle staff striking?
Medical attendants

The Imperial School of Medical caretakers (RCN) says its individuals ought to have a 19% compensation rise.

The public authority says this is unreasonably expensive and no compensation rise near that has been advertised:

NHS staff in Britain and Ribs - including attendants - have previously been given a normal increment of 4.75%. The most minimal paid were ensured an ascent of no less than £1,400
In Northern Ireland, medical attendants will get a similar increment, which will be predated

In Scotland, a compensation offer averaging 7.5% for NHS staff has been acknowledged by certain associations, however, dismissed by RCN and RCM individuals
The RCN says normal compensation for attendants has previously fallen by 6% somewhere in the range of 2011 and 2021, whenever expansion is considered.

The association said it would set a 48-hour cutoff time after the strike closes for the public authority to examine pay.

With no arrangement, more activity will be declared for the new year. The RCN has around 300,000 individuals - about 66% of NHS medical attendants.

Does the typical medical caretaker procure £34,000 per year?
Could each 1% ascent to medical attendants' compensation cost £700m?
Emergency vehicle staff

They likewise need above-expansion pay rises, yet have not set a particular figure.

Associations contend that any proposition should be sufficiently high to forestall an emergency vehicle staff enlistment emergency. In Scotland, two associations have proactively acknowledged a superior compensation proposition of 7.5%.

The UK government, in any case, says pay ascends for rescue vehicle laborers and attendants were concluded by autonomous compensation audit bodies.

How much are medical caretakers paid?

The beginning compensation for a medical caretaker in Britain is simply over £27,000 per year. This is the lower part of pay band five of the NHS contract, known as Plan for Change.

Staff, for example, medical services partners, watchmen, and cleaners are in lower pay groups.

Under the agreement, the staff is qualified for in-the-work increments inside their compensation band.

Diagram showing pay groups
A medical caretaker with four years' experience could hope to procure nearly £33,000 - the top finish of pay band five.

Expert medical attendants can make up to £47,000.

The most senior medical attendant experts can acquire up to almost £55,000.

CHAPTER NINE: Winter of discontent.

Gigantic strikes are making confusion in emergency clinics and halts at travel center points, as walkouts by firemen, things controllers, paramedics, driving analysts, migration officials, transport drivers, development laborers, mail transporters, and rail route guides mount. The public has been cautioned to keep away from train travel on Christmas Eve.

The English government is presently planning to activate 1,200 armed force troops to drive ambulances over special times of the year. Government workers from different offices will be acquired to take a look at visas at line intersections, if fundamental.

During the most awful long periods of the Covid pandemic, a huge number of conventional Britons, close by Top state leader Boris Johnson (likewise gone), remained on their doorsteps during brutal lockdowns to bang pots and dish and applaud for Public Wellbeing Administration laborers, hailing them as cutting edge legends.

Presently the medical attendants are saying they need more than commendation. They are worn out, exhausted, and came up short on, they say, and believe a genuine raise should stay aware of expansion, which has topped 10%.

"They're exploiting us," said Rachel Ambrose, 40, a psychological well-being medical caretaker who works with kids and teens in Oxford. "We don't look for a lavish way of life. We're medical attendants. We simply need to cover our bills. We need heat."

Ambrose said that the medical caretakers are "started up, we're, still up in the air," and that these strikes "will proceed because they are disregarding us."

She highlighted staffing deficiencies at the NHS that sabotage patient consideration and have medical caretakers at a limit. Days off have taken off since the pandemic — thus medical attendants leaving the calling or moving to another country.

U.K. attendants, battling to cover bills, say a strike is for the eventual fate of medical services

England's general well-being framework is short 50,000 attendants. A big part of all fresh recruits today come from abroad because the U.K. either can't prepare enough at home or pays excessively little to draw in new specialists. Brexit likewise has stemmed the "free development" stream of medical caretakers from Eastern Europe to England.

The public authority says the typical attendant's compensation is presently 35,600 pounds ($43,300). New medical attendants are saved money; experienced medical caretakers with particular abilities are paid more; additional time likewise helps pay rates.

Attendants procure higher wages in the US, Canada, Australia, Ireland, Germany, and Spain. English attendants, however, are paid more than their partners in France and Italy.

Following one of the most awful long stretches of strikes in late English history, Head of the state Rishi Sunak's new government is as yet declining to find a spot at the table with the associations, calling the compensation expands "exorbitant" and cautioning that the public authority should hang tight on wages to hold expansion in line.

The public authority upholds a humble increase in salary for rescue vehicle teams and medical caretakers – as suggested by free compensation survey bodies – of around 4.75 percent. The medical caretakers association is requesting a 19 percent increment.

Sunak's representative on Monday let columnists know that "it would be unreliable to push ahead with twofold digit pay grants."

England's trains come to a standstill in the greatest rail strike in 30 years

However, Sunak and his administration priests are discovering that it is one thing to battle the rail line laborers and their "association supervisors," as the public authority brands them, and everyone more to battle the attendants. The rail route strikes make disappointing growls for metropolitan suburbanites and occasion explorers — which are featured by the counter association tabloids. The medical caretakers, then again, are respected. A YouGov survey this month found that 64% of Britons upheld the medical caretakers' strike.

On Monday, Sunak assembled a crisis bureau conference to shape intends to make a big difference for the country's crucial public administrations, with the military on backup.

Around 10,000 emergency vehicle laborers in Britain and Ridges are set to picket Wednesday. Individuals from the Illustrious School of Nursing association left Thursday and made a beeline for the picket lines again Tuesday.

Attendants who work in trauma centers have remained at work, yet medical clinics are attempting to keep up with staffing for fundamental consideration. Numerous standard strategies, tests, non-crisis medical procedures, and different therapies have been deferred.

A few survivors of the coronary episode or stroke are standing by close to 60 minutes on normal for ambulances – contrasted and the 18-minute objective.

At area specialists' workplaces, where most patients see their overall professional and medical caretakers, the staffs portray a framework in an emergency because of ongoing underfunding and laborer deficiencies.

Anthony Johnson, 29, a heart nurturer in Leeds, is among those supporting the choice by the Illustrious School of Nursing to leave without precedent for its 106-year history.

"We have not had pay rises that meet expansion. That is the reason you see attendants going to food banks and the number of opportunities has radically expanded," he said. "We have horrible attendant-to-patient proportions. Our clinical rules are one medical caretaker to eight patients, yet we never buy and that's what large meet. Actually, it's one medical caretaker to 13 patients, so it's continually hazardous and seriously jeopardizes patients."

He prefers working in England and will remain. In any case, many are looking abroad, he cautioned.

"We're preparing medical attendants for sending out, typically to Canada, Australia, and New Zealand ... where attendants can make an extra 10,000 pounds [$12,200]," Johnson said. "As opposed to putting resources into our staff, the U.K. government is taking medical attendants from different regions of the planet. They are cutting compensation and allowing that to occur."

Julia Patterson, the organizer behind Each Specialist, a mission bunch addressing 1,200 U.K. doctors, said her PCPs are "truly strong and will arrange to guard patients without medical caretakers. They should buckle down, yet they support their partners doing this."

She noticed that specialists, as well, are being balloted to check whether they could strike in the new year.

"Individuals are kicking the bucket due to a disappointment in general well-being," Patterson said.

'We can't adapt any longer': Frantic and with next to no other choice, these are the NHS attendants headed to strike
"As time continues - sadly on the off chance that this administration doesn't address us and doesn't get into a room - I'm anxious about the possibility that this will raise,"

In the meantime, one week from now will be "extremely difficult" for the well-being administration during a new flood of strikes by the two medical caretakers and emergency vehicle laborers, break CEO of NHS Suppliers said.

What precisely is the strike about? We should separate it:

What have attendants been advertised?
Recently, medical caretakers were offered a compensation rise for working out at around 4 to 5 percent alongside other public area laborers.

Most full-time nurture in the NHS would get a compensation increment of around £1,400. New nursing staff, in any case, would see beginning compensation ascend by 5.5 percent to £27,055.

The wellbeing secretary, Steve Barclay, said the public authority was adhering to the proposals of the free NHS Pay Audit Body.

A large number of medical caretakers are striking

What is it that medical attendants need?

The Illustrious School of Nursing (RCN) depicted the 4% essential boost in salary for most medical caretakers as a "grave stumble by clergymen" when it was declared in summer.

Its overall secretary, Pat Cullen, said at that point: "Living expenses are rising but they have implemented other genuine terms pay cut on nursing staff," she said. "It will push more medical caretakers and nursing support laborers out of the calling."

The expansion has been rising above the previous year, with the most recent figures putting it at 10.7 percent.

The RCN has been requiring a compensation ascend at 5% above expansion. Notwithstanding, the association has shown it would acknowledge a lower offer.

The association has contended that low compensation is driving "persistent understaffing" which endangers patients and leaves nursing staff exhausted, coming up short on and underestimated.

In Scotland, RCN individuals are being counseled on a reconsidered pay offer from the Scottish government.

And talks?

Last-ditch converses with keep away from strikes separated for the current week.

Ms. Cullen said strikes would go on after the well-being secretary would not examine pay. The public authority said it would keep on connecting on non-pay related issues and has said the compensation rise requested by the RCN was excessively expensive.

After the principal walkout on Thursday, Bringing down Road has said there are "no plans" to take a gander at the compensation bargain for medical caretakers.

What else are medical caretakers talking about?

As well as pay, medical caretakers have told The Free they are striking over working circumstances and understaffing. Some said security has been undermined by deficiencies.

"The principal reason we're doing this is that we go into our responsibility to care for others and we're not doing that very well right now given the absence of staffing, the absence of interest into nursing," one London nurture said.

Others have told The Free medical caretakers were attempting to manage the cost of fundamentals and were being driven away from the calling or work through yearly leave.

Up to 100 000 nursing staff across the UK left in the first of two days of strike activity on 15 December, after the public authority wouldn't move on pay requests, contending that it would imply "removing cash from forefront administrations."

The primary strike day came after under portion of Britain's NHS trusts (102 of 215) arrived at the half-turnout edge required for strike activity. All nursing staff in Northern Ireland and everything except one of the wellbeing sheets in Ribs additionally met the threshold.1

A subsequent strike is made arrangements for 20 December, which will be trailed by a more drawn-out time of activity on the off chance that legislatures keep on denying formal compensation exchanges or on the other hand if pays talks don't bring about a palatable result, said the Illustrious School of Nursing.

The Fair Compensation for Nursing effort is requiring a boost in salary that is 5% above expansion (estimated by the retail cost file (RPI)), which would presently mean a 17.6% compensation rise. The public authority has said this would cost around £9bn, as inspire would likewise have to cover all staff on the Plan for Change contract, which ...

The very first public strike of NHS attendants starts today (15 December) after pastors would not haggle on pay.

Attendants in Britain, Grains, and Northern Ireland will likewise leave on 20 December, following cases by the public authority that it can't alter compensations proposed by the free compensation body for NHS staff.

Associations had proposed to cancel the activity if another compensation arrangement could be reached, and the Regal School of Nursing has blamed the public authority for "picking strike activity". An arrangement was struck in Scotland that deflected strikes recently.

Direct activity will happen on all sides of the NHS in the three leftover districts, including rescue vehicle administrations, recommending there has been an emotional change in mindset among well-being laborers throughout the last year.

We hear reports of the NHS in an emergency, clinics running at the limit, and perilously low staffing levels. Yet, without working inside these administrations, it's difficult to genuinely comprehend what this resembles for staff, and the patients these staff are giving a valiant effort to focus on.

What staff is seeing direct is a horrendous breakdown of administrations that have left us with opportunities hitting 135,000 and patients at serious risk. We frantically need to zero in on the maintenance of staff: without tending to that, we get no opportunity of handling the overabundance of 7,000,000 patients. Tragically, neither the public authority nor resistance truly carries maintenance into the discussion, since that would mean putting pay rebuilding on the plan.

In a new overview by the GMB association, one of every three rescue vehicle staff said they had been engaged with a defer that had brought about an individual kicking the bucket. This is a frightening measurement, and only one of numerous that the public authority ought to be viewing undeniably more in a serious way.

Staff are not ready to remain with their hands behind their backs while the NHS is torn and separated before our eyes

What we are currently seeing are progressively outrageous assaults from the conservative press and pundits endeavoring to vilify us, and coerce us into leaving our battle for what we are owed.

Be that as it may, as I remarked to a partner, nothing they can say regarding us will be essentially as terrible as the thing staff is seeing every day of the week. Things can't go on as they are, and staff is not ready to remain with their hands behind their backs while the NHS is torn and separated before our eyes.

I have filled in as an NHS nurturer for quite a long time. I love my work. However, my compensation, and that of my partners, has been purposely dissolved for north of 10 years, for certain laborers up to 29% more regrettable off in genuine terms. What we are left with is a gathering of laborers worrying about the whole concern of guarding patients, while the public authority disavows any liability or responsibility for the condition of the help inside which they work.

These are the staff who wind up skipping breaks, staying at work past 40 hours free of charge, offering back their yearly pass on to earn enough to get by, and resting in their vehicles as they can't manage the cost of fuel to and from work - and eventually stopping, as the ethical injury of conveying unacceptable consideration isn't maintainable.

We ought to be in every way joined in our shock. While this is a modern question about pay, the quarrel is over a great deal more. During the pandemic, we saw the overwhelming effect of emphatically expanded requests on an NHS that has been stripped deep down. We can't allow this to repeat.

For this reason, we are taking our battle to this administration and standing up for ourselves, however for our families and networks, and the fate of the NHS. So when the opportunity arrives, it will kindly join NHS staff on the picket lines.

Without activity now, there will be no NHS passed on to battle for.

In the US, there has been a persistent discussion between the people who favor aggregate expecting medical caretakers and the individuals who accept it isn't proficient. Moreover, the discussion about whether medical attendants ought to strike has been longstanding and go on today. The individuals who go against medical caretakers striking frequently express that they are leaving their patients and that it isn't moral, although government regulation requires a 10-day strike notice so the executives can make patient consideration game plans. The American Medical caretakers Affiliation (ANA) has upheld the right of medical caretakers to strike if all else fails and after cautious thought of each variable. This help has partitioned the participation of ANA and the nursing calling, even though the strikes have been utilized sparingly and actually by attendants in this nation; thus the discussion proceeds.

Patient well-being can't be ensured, industry body says
Striking medical attendants looking for above-expansion pay increment
Rescue vehicle laborers to leave Wednesday
Clergymen will not examine pay

Around 100,000 medical caretakers picketed on Tuesday for the second opportunity in seven days as their association gave a final proposal to the public authority to answer pay requests in something like 48 hours or face one more round of modern activity in January.

Promotion · Look to proceed

Rescue vehicle staff in Britain and Ribs are set to stick to this same pattern on Wednesday and Dec. 28, leaving those with everything except the most hazardous circumstances to make their specific manner to an emergency clinic.

"We can't ensure patient security, we can't stay away from gambles in that frame of mind of this modern activity," Matthew Taylor, CEO of the NHS Confederation which addresses public well-being administration associations, told BBC Radio.

"We are stressed over the dangers tomorrow however with the chance of additional strikes creating as winter unfurls ... we are going into an extremely perilous time. To this end, we are increasing considerably more our call to the public authority and the worker's organizations to attempt to track down an approach to settling this debate."

The strike by attendants is uncommon in the Regal School of Nursing (RCN) association's 106-year history, yet it says it must choose between limited options as the taking off typical cost for most everyday items leaves laborers battling to earn enough to get by.

The RCN says its individuals' genuine term profit has fallen by 6% somewhat recently and has required compensation transcend the RPI pace of expansion, which remained at 14% in November.

The public authority granted medical attendants around 4% overall, on the proposal of an autonomous compensation survey body, and has declined to examine pay further. Head of the state Rishi Sunak says the medical caretakers' requests are unreasonably expensive.

"I will haggle with him anytime to quit nursing staff and patients going into the new year confronting such vulnerability," RCN head Pat Cullen said.

Medical caretakers strike outside College School Emergency clinic in London

[1/11] NHS medical caretakers hold bulletins during a strike, amid a question with the public authority over pay, outside College School Clinic in London, England December 20, 2022.

"Yet, if this administration isn't ready to make the best choice, we'll have no real option except to go on in January."

The strikes are coming down on medical care arrangements in the state-supported Public Wellbeing Administration when it is extended by staff deficiencies and record overabundances because of Coronavirus delays.

An emergency clinic in southern Britain and the South East Coast Rescue vehicle Administration both said on Tuesday they had proclaimed a basic episode because of outrageous tensions in their administrations.

"Our individuals are burnt out on going to work consistently and at times, spending the entirety of their shift sat on an emergency vehicle outside an A&E division with a similar patient," Rachel Harrison, GMB association public administration public secretary, told a panel of legislators.

"We've had models where our individuals have timed off toward the finish of one shift to return the next day to the very persistent being on that emergency vehicle."

The military has been placed on backup to assist with driving ambulances and pastors are meeting with associations on Tuesday to talk about which crises ambulances will in any case answer, during media reports those enduring coronary failures or strokes probably won't qualify.

Lady Rose James has been in the NHS for a considerable length of time. She said now it is "significantly more challenging for attendants to come into the positions after they removed the bursary".

"So learner medical attendants need to burn through cash preparing and for what? To be paid at times not exactly if you worked in a café. There's something wrong with that. We want to hold our splendid medical caretakers."

Research nurture Glyn Fletcher works with stroke patients and has been in the NHS for quite a long time. He said: "I love my work. I was very disturbed when I decided in favor of the strike activity.

"It's with overwhelming sadness that I am around here today. I wasn't even certain assuming I planned to come to the picket line. However, we need to. Nursing is an emergency and pay is a major piece of that.

"In any case, we additionally need the public authority to perceive that without medical attendants the NHS can't work."

Appointee ward chief Catherine Hughes-McGreal said she needs the public authority to "sit up and pay attention to us".

"We have deficient staffing numbers and it's not manageable. This all boils down to patient security. Not a solitary one of us needs to be over here yet we must choose between limited options.

"Here and there we're overextended to such an extent that we are stressed that slip-ups will be made and individuals will kick the bucket. It's horrendous."

Nursing partner Alison Kamperis said the public authority is "making an honest effort to wreck the NHS".

"Indeed, we need better compensation. Be that as it may, it's not just about paying. Keeping our splendid attendants in this profession is tied in with attempting. We are depleted and flattened and it's no time like the present the public authority gave us a fair arrangement."

Nurture Dave Carr has worked in the NHS for quite a long time. Talking from London, he said: "We can't convey ensure patient security any longer.

"We can't ensure the occupation is just about as protected as it ought to be. We want a compensation rise for cash in our pockets, however, to hold staff to keep staff we want compensation to ascend to save the NHS."

Ethna Vaughan said the "entire NHS is feeling the squeeze and everybody feels it".

She added: "The foolish mentality of the public authority and not paying medical caretakers enough means in the long haul, it's hard to get attendants into the calling and it's challenging for medical attendants who need to remain because they can't stand to."

England is confronting an influx of modern activity this colder time of year, with strikes devastating the rail organization and postal help, and air terminals preparing for disturbance over Christmas.

Expansion running at over 10%, followed by pay offers of around 4%, is stirring up strains among associations and managers.

Of the relative multitude of strikes, however, it will be seeing medical caretakers on picket lines that will be the stand-apart picture for some Britons this colder time of year.

Shocking DAY

"What a terrible day. This is a terrible day for nursing, it is an unfortunate day for patients, patients in medical clinics like this, and it is a sad day for individuals of this general public and our NHS," Pat Cullen, the top of the Regal School of Nursing

(RCN) association, told the BBC on a picket line.

The generally appreciated nursing calling shut down pieces of the NHS, which since its establishment in 1948 has created irreplaceable asset status for being free at the reason behind use, hitting medical services arrangement when it is extended in winter and with accumulations at record levels because of Coronavirus delays.

Wellbeing clergyman Steve Barclay said it was profoundly unfortunate that the strike was going for it.

"I've been working across government and with surgeons outside the public area to guarantee safe staffing levels - however, I truly do stay worried about the gamble that pauses dramatically to patients," he said.

MORE STRIKES AHEAD?

The modern activity by attendants on Dec. 15 and Dec. 20 is extraordinary in the English nursing association's 106-year history, yet the RCN says it must choose between limited options as laborers battle to earn barely enough to get by.

Attendants need a compensation ascent of 5% in addition to the expansion, contending they have experienced 10 years of genuine terms cuts and that low compensation implies staff deficiencies and perilous consideration for patients. The public authority says their interest would compare to a 19% climb.

The public authority has would not talk about pay, which Cullen said raised the possibility of additional strikes into the following year.

"Nothing is changing and I've been in nursing for a considerable length of time and all I can see is a consistent decrease in confidence," she told Reuters.

In Belfast, passing vehicles sounded their horns on the side of the attendants accumulated on picket lines beneath frosty temperatures outside the Regal Victoria Medical clinic.

"I didn't go with this choice delicately ... I concluded the time had come to say 'enough'," said Louise Mitchell, who has been a medical caretaker for quite some time.

"We don't maintain that patients should experience any longer. Patient consideration is experiencing the entire week in this country since there isn't an adequate number of assets in the wellbeing administration."

The public authority in Scotland kept away from a nursing strike by holding chats on pay, a result that the RCN had expected in Britain, Grains, and Northern Ireland.

Yet, the public authority has said it can't bear to pay more than the 4-5% proposed to medical attendants, which was suggested by a free body, and that further boosts in compensation would mean removing cash from cutting-edge administrations.

Some therapy regions were absolved from the strike, the RCN has said, including chemotherapy, dialysis, and escalated care.

Surveying in front of the nursing strike recommended a greater part of Britons upheld the activity.

CONCLUSION

The fight for fair pay for nurses is one that has been ongoing for decades and it is still far from being resolved. Although there are some positive developments, such as the implementation of fair pay systems and higher salaries in some states, it is clear that there is still a long way to go. Nurses are still underpaid and undervalued compared to other professions and they are facing an uphill battle to get the pay they deserve. They are not just fighting for fair pay, but for respect and recognition.

The fight for fair pay for nurses is a fight for all of us. We can all help by supporting legislation and initiatives that ensure fair pay for nurses and advocating for better pay and better working conditions. We must also speak up and show our support for our nurses who are on the front lines of healthcare. We must make sure that our elected officials understand the importance of investing in our nurses and that they are paid fairly for the hard work they put in every day.

The fight for fair pay for nurses is an important one, and it is one that will take time and effort to win. But if we all come together and commit to it, then we can make a real difference and ensure that nurses get the pay and respect they deserve.

Our striking nurses have already made significant progress in their fight for fair pay. However, there is still a long way to go. It is up to us to make sure that the fight for fair pay for nurses does not end here. Let us come together and make sure that our nurses get the pay and respect they deserve.

www.ingramcontent.com/pod-product-compliance
Lightning Source LLC
LaVergne TN
LVHW050322160826
845677LV00014B/3513

9798370832543